A Yoga Journey Through India

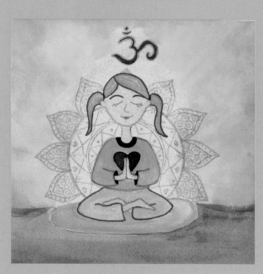

Library of Congress Cataloging-in-Publication Data Available

ISBN: 978-1-7751434-1-3

Published by Art Mindfulness and Creativity
www.artmindfulnessandcreativity.com

Dedication:

For my daughter Ella, you teach me how to enjoy the precious moments of life and to be mindful each day. For all the students I have ever taught, may you find joy in the mindful moments of life and for all of my fellow yogi's I love to practice and learn from you.

AMC

Namaste, today we are going on a journey to India. Namaste is used in India to greet others as well as a way to open and close your yoga practice. India is on the continent of Asia.

Easy Pose/ Sukhasana
Take a breath in and lengthen your spine nice and tall. Sit criss cross with your hands at prayer center and take a few centering breaths.

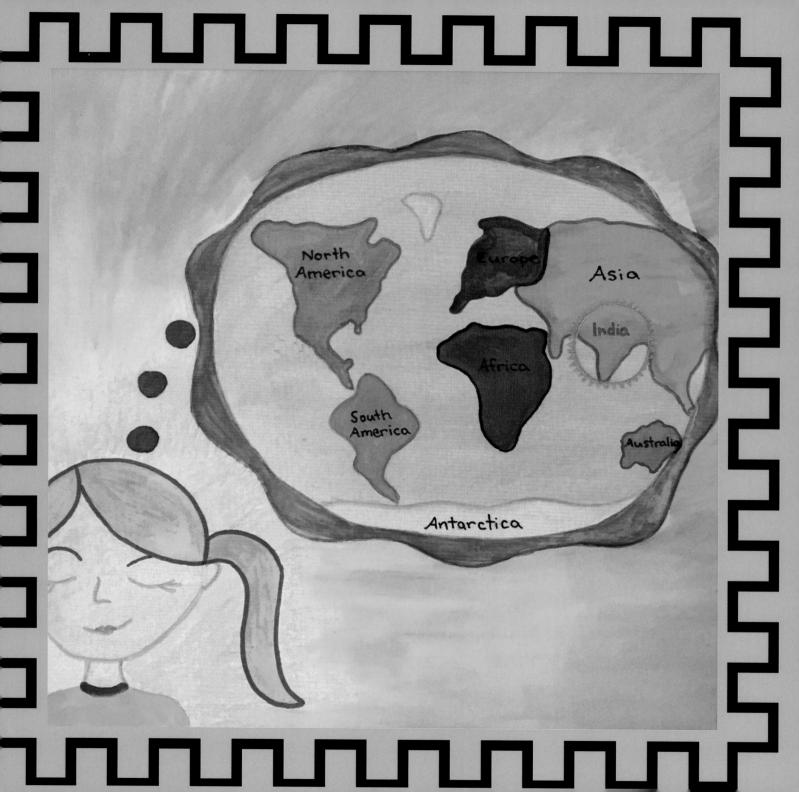

Did you know there are many different animals in India? There is everything from the roaring Bengal Tiger to the grazing Water Buffalo.

Cat Cow/ Marjariasana
Lean forward onto your hands and knees into a tabletop position. Arch your back up to the sky like an angry tiger and do your best tiger roar. Lower your belly and tilt your head up to the sky to be a water buffalo. Arch your back and be a bengal tiger, lower your belly for your water buffalo. Breathe out as you arch your back into a tiger and inhale as you lower your belly and lift your head into a water buffalo.
Repeat at least three more times.

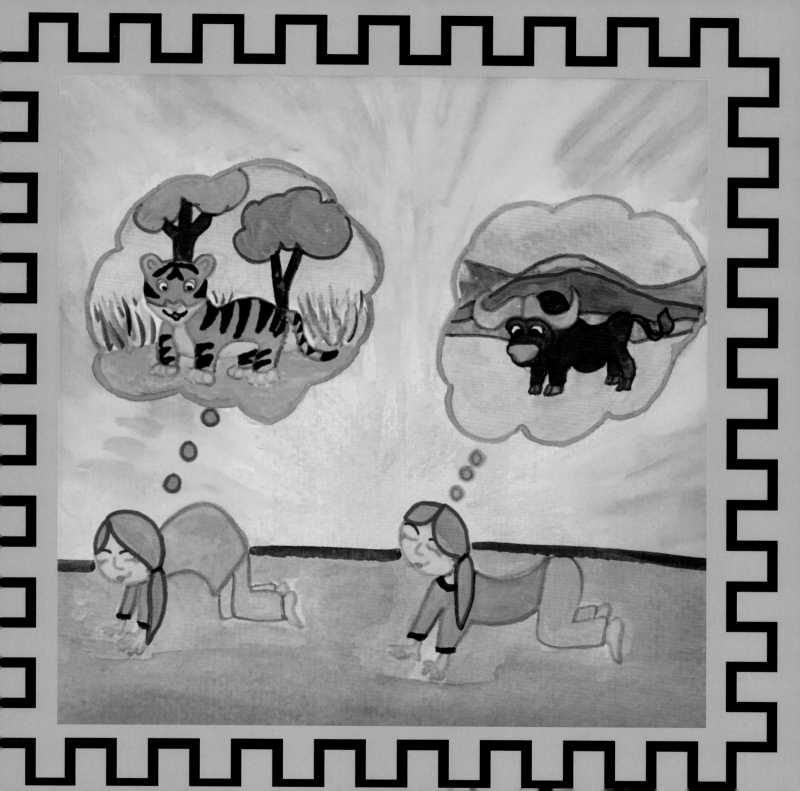

The Himalayan Mountain range passes through the northern most tip of India. This is the youngest and highest mountain range in the world. You will fly over it to get to India

Down Dog/ Adho Mukha Svanasana
Push your hips up to the sky like a great big mountain. Stretch out your legs and feel them grounding you to the earth. When you feel ready look forward step to the top edge of your mat. Half lift, breath in and lower down. Bend your knees slightly and reach all the way up to the sky, lower your arms into prayer centre. Stand tall, feet parallel, chest lifted. Flex your toes to ground your legs. Press your palms together at your chest.

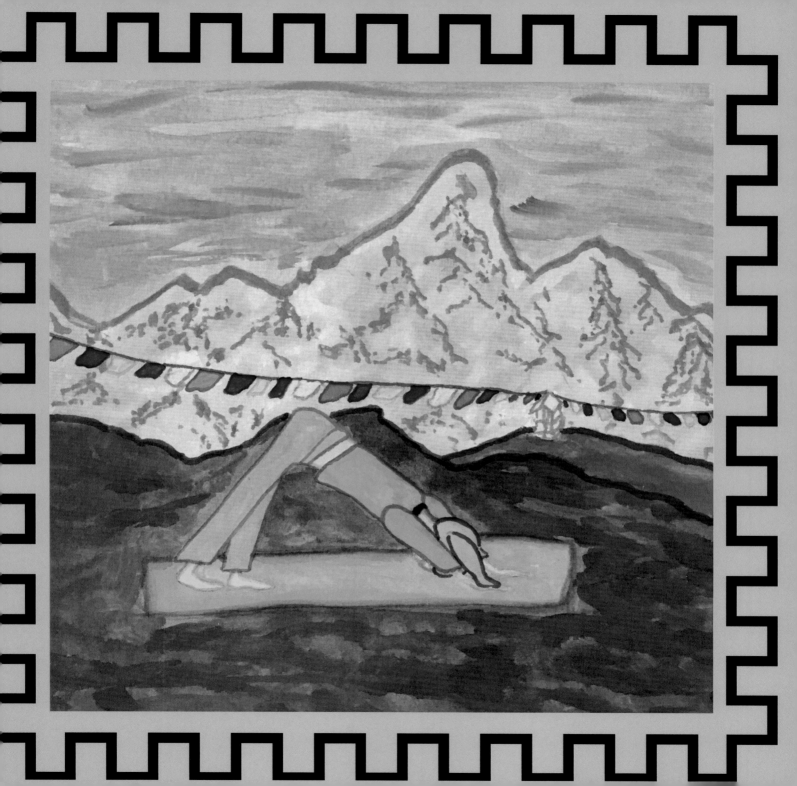

It is a long flight from North America to India. To fly there we will have to make a stop in Europe to refuel then head on to New Delhi. New Delhi is India's capital city.

Airplane/ Dekasana
Stand with feet parallel and under hips. Breathe, focus and stretch your right leg back. Tip forward until you are parallel with the floor. Spread your arms out like wings and fly. Lower your right leg and stand tall. Stand with feet parallel and under hips. Breathe, focus and stretch your left leg back. Tip forward until you are parallel with the floor. Spread your arms out like wings and fly.

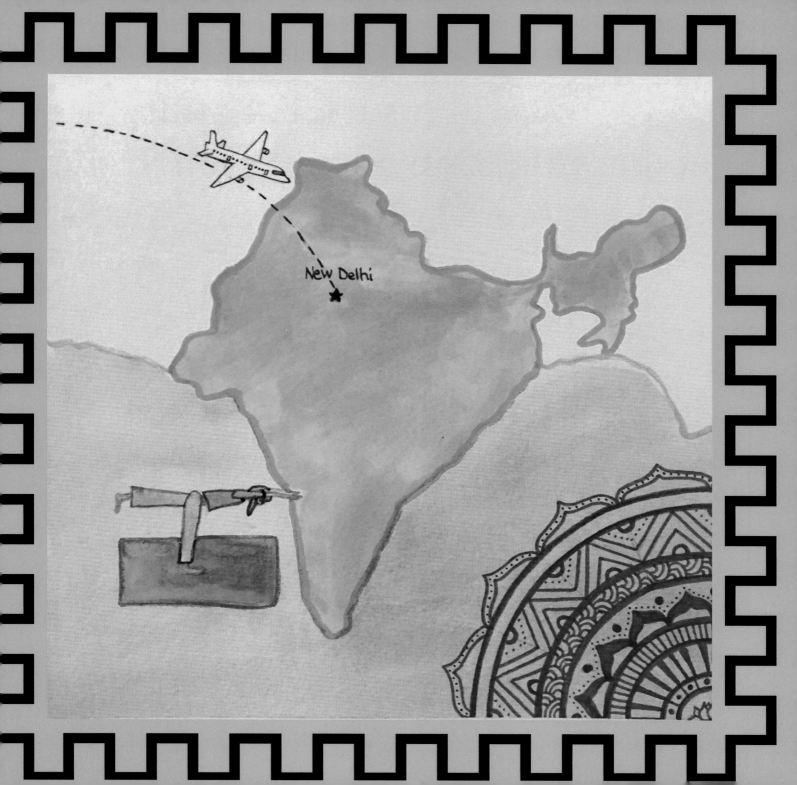

You will need trust and communication to get through the busy streets of New Delhi. There are 21.5 million people living in this bustling metropolis.

Warrior Friends/ Virabhadrasana
Pair up with a partner on one mat. Face each other right foot to right foot. Step your left leg back and bend your right knees. Link hands left to right, right to left. Twist open and deepen the stretch. Focus on your partner's eyes and see if you can communicate without words. Release your hands step back to the top of your mat facing each other. Step your right leg back and bend your left knee. Link hands right to left and left to right. Twist open and deepen the stretch. Again focus on your partner's eyes. Release your hands and step back to the top of your mat facing each other.

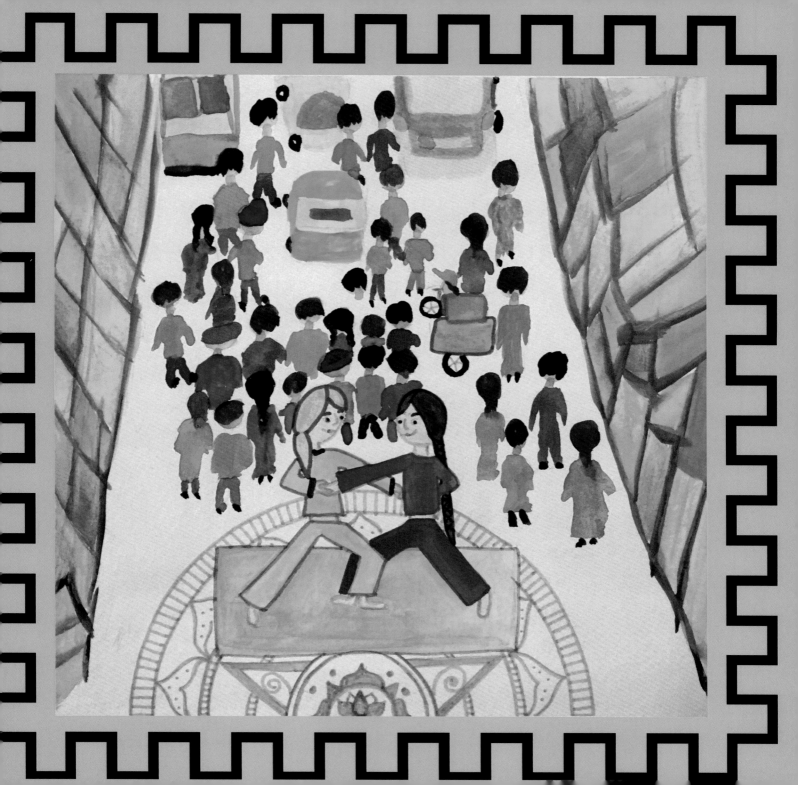

Let's get on a rickshaw and tour the city. A rickshaw is a two or three wheel passenger cart usually pulled by a man. On our tour we may come across many famous structures like the Red Fort, the Qutab Minar (which is the tallest brick minaret in the world), and the Bahai Temple.

Back to Back Chair/ Utkatasana

Turn around so that your backs are together. Sit down back-to-back on the floor. Bend your knees, feet flat and hook elbows. Push into each other's backs and press up to bent knees as though you are sitting in a chair, supporting each other with your back. Hold your chair pose for a few moments then press all the way up to standing.

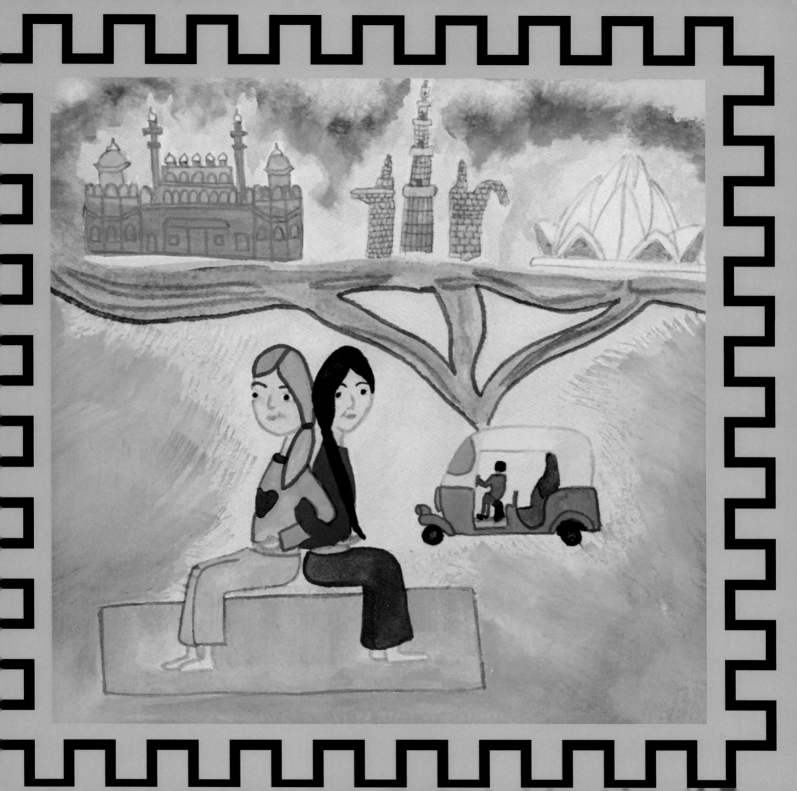

The Bahai temple is a special temple, made out of white marble shaped petals. It proclaims unity of all people and religions, everyone is welcome to worship here. Also, it is known as the Lotus Temple because it is shaped like a lotus flower

Face to Face Chair/ Utkatasana

Turn and face your partner and hold your partner by both wrists. Lean back so that you are both supporting each other. While you lean back bend your knees until they are at a 90 degree angle. Hold your chair pose for a few breaths, focusing on supporting each other. When ready straighten your legs to standing.

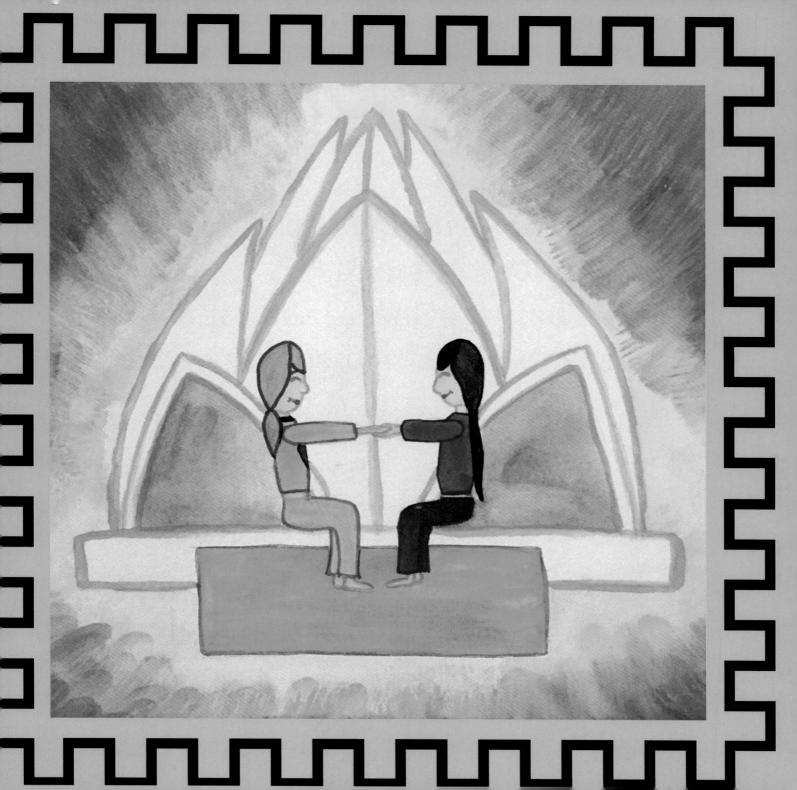

Moving along on our tour, to the city of Agra. Here you will find one of the New Seven Wonders of the World, the Taj Mahal. Construction of the Taj Mahal began in 1632. It means 'Crown Palace' and was built by Shah Jahan in memory of his wife. It is a mausoleum made of white marble.

Partner Open Heart/ Anahata

Stand behind your partner so that one of you is facing the others back. Get the partner in the front to reach back with their arms. Hold your partner's wrists. Let your partner arch and lean forward. Hold your partner as they stretch fully forward. Make sure they are fully supported so they do not fall forward. Open up your chest and your heart to all of the love and acceptance in the world. Allow your partner to stand back up and switch positions.

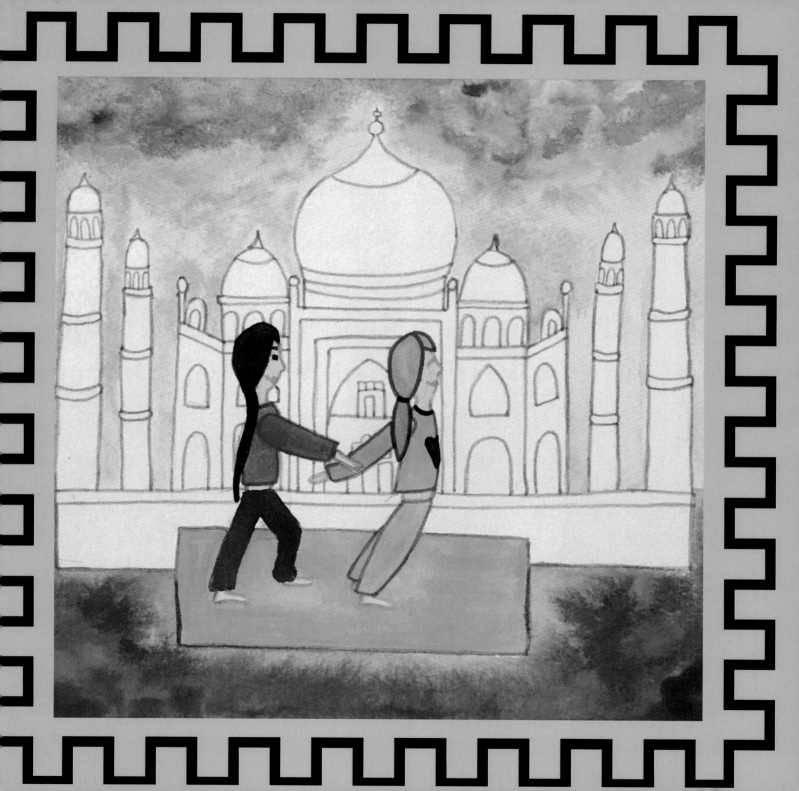

Man I am tired of being in the busy cities, let's head out to the countryside. Did you know that elephants live in India? Elephants are actually a very special animal. They even have celebrations once a year in Jaipur city called the Elephant festival. It is celebrated during Holi, the Festival of Colour.

Elephant Breath/ Pranayama (Breathing)
Stand with your feet wide apart, link your hands and dangle your arms in front of you like an elephant trunk. Inhale through your nose as you raise your arms high above your head and lean back. Exhale through your mouth as you swing your arms down and through your legs. Repeat this 5 times.

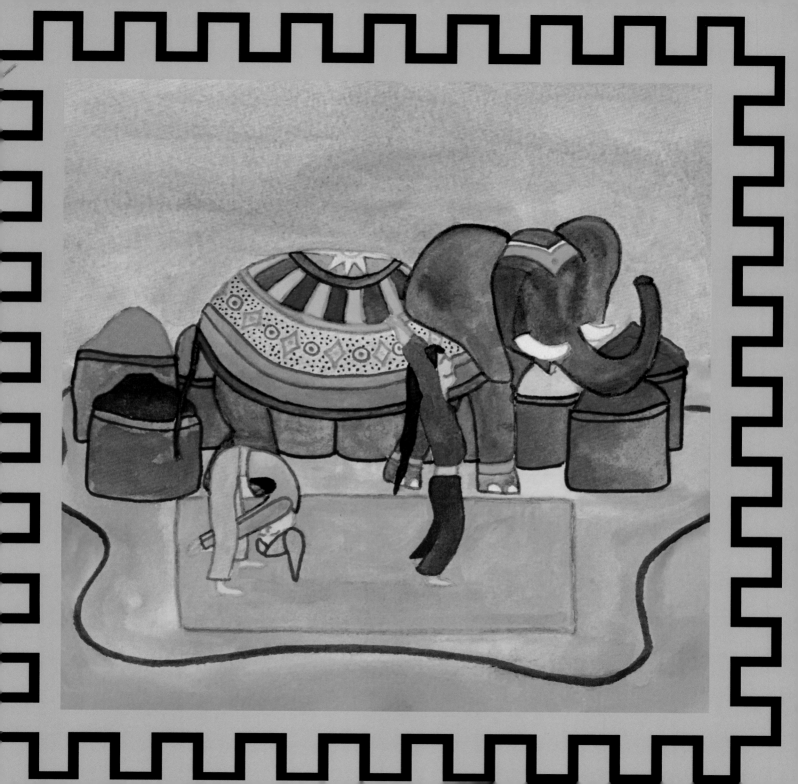

Another unique animal is the River Dolphin, it calls the Ganges and Brahamaputra Rivers home. These rivers flow through one of the world's most densely populated areas. The River Dolphin is threatened by removal of river water, pollution and entanglement in fishing nets.

Dolphin Pose/ Ardha Pincha Mayurasana
Stand at the top of your mat. Reach up to the sky, breath in, exhale place your palms on the mat and step back. Lower your knees and elbows to the mat, clasp your hands together at the top of your mat. Push up on to your toes and press your legs straight. Walk your feet towards your elbows.

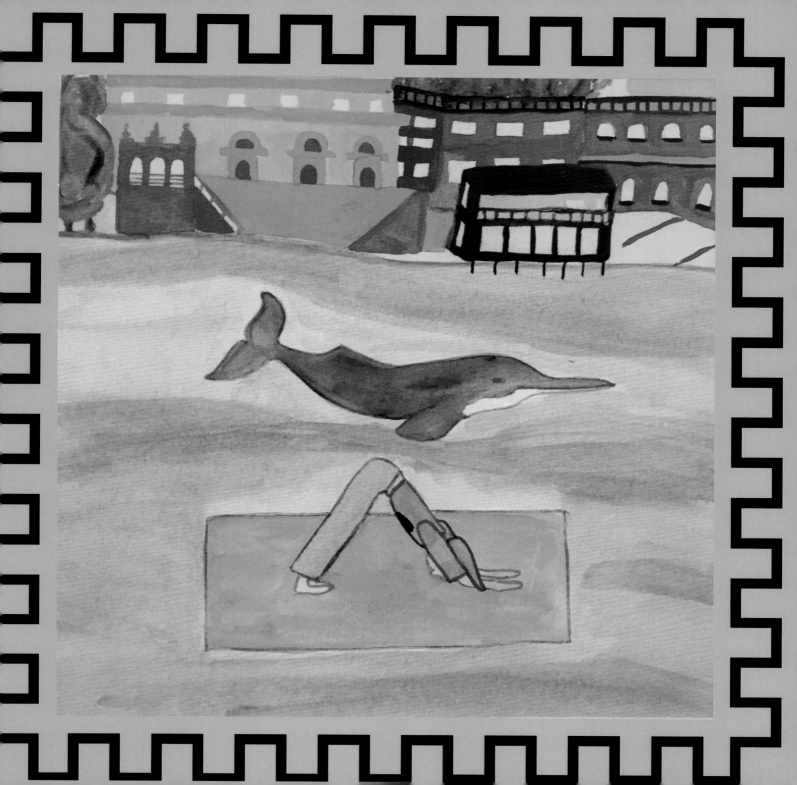

Let's go for a boat ride down the Ganges River. This is a very sacred river to people who are Hindu. It is also a very polluted river, and is considered to be the 5th most polluted river in the world. It is also the third largest river by discharge.

Boat Pose/ Navasana
Sit back on to your bottom with your feet out in front of you, bend your knees in and place your feet on the ground. Put your arms out in front of you and reach for your knees. If you feel supported, lift and point your toes. Stretch out your arms and balance on your bottom.

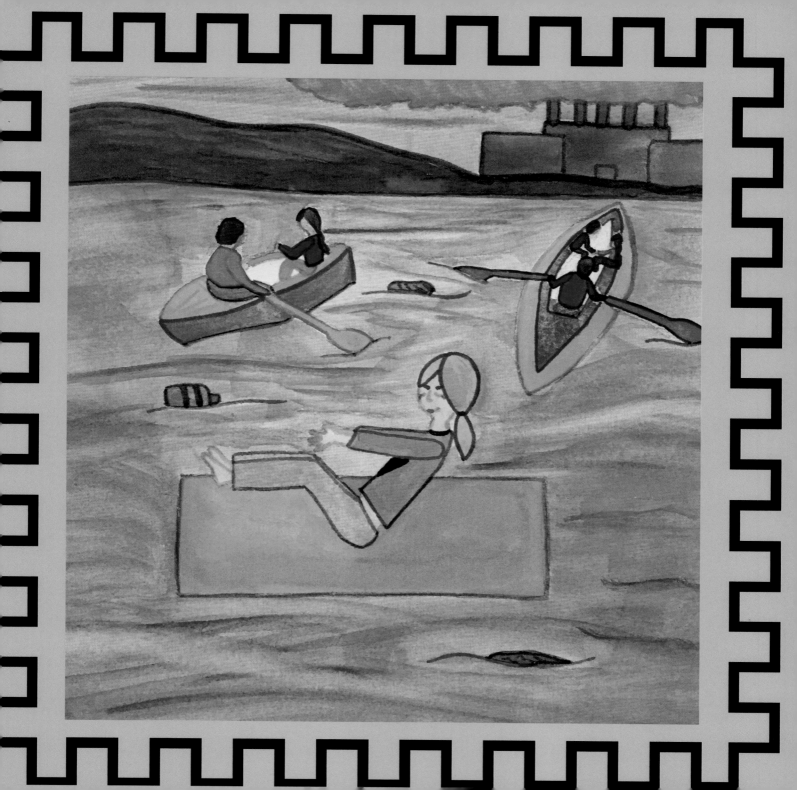

It has been a busy trip, lets relax with the current of the water. Imagine the Ganges River flowing from the Himalayan Mountains, across the Gangetic Plains of Northern India into Bangladesh and eventually emptying into the Bay of Bengal. This long flowing river provides water to about 40% of India's population, serving an estimated 500 million people.

Forward Fold/ Paschimottanasana

Stretch your feet straight out in front of you and sit tall. Press your hands down and lengthen your back. Reach your hands to your feet and hold your calves, ankles or toes. Stretch your chest out over your legs. As you hold the pose imagine you are a gentle river, you are long and fluid, breathe in and out and relax into your fold.

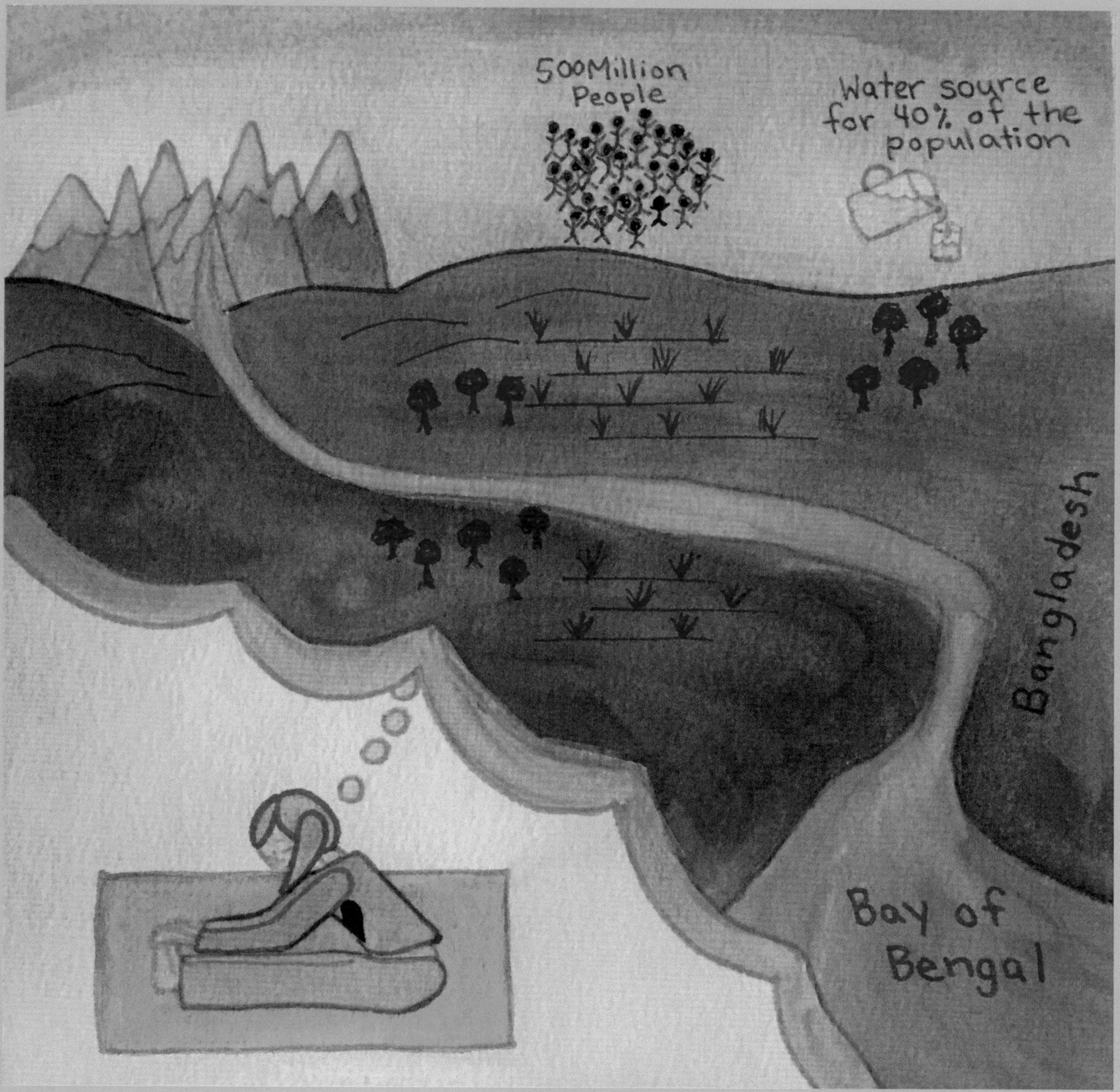
500Million People
Water source for 40% of the population
Bangladesh
Bay of Bengal

India is home to not only animals and people but many insects as well. It is believed to be home to over 1200 species of butterflies. Imagine you are a beautiful butterfly flapping your wings. Allow your wings to slowly lift you off and travel all the way home.

Butterfly/ Badhakonasana

Bend your knees in and touch the outer edges of the feet together, allow your knees to fall open to the sides like a book. Interlace your hands around your feet. Press the thighs and shins down toward the floor as you bend forward, pause and breathe. Sit up, stretch your legs out straight and slowly lay down on to your mat.

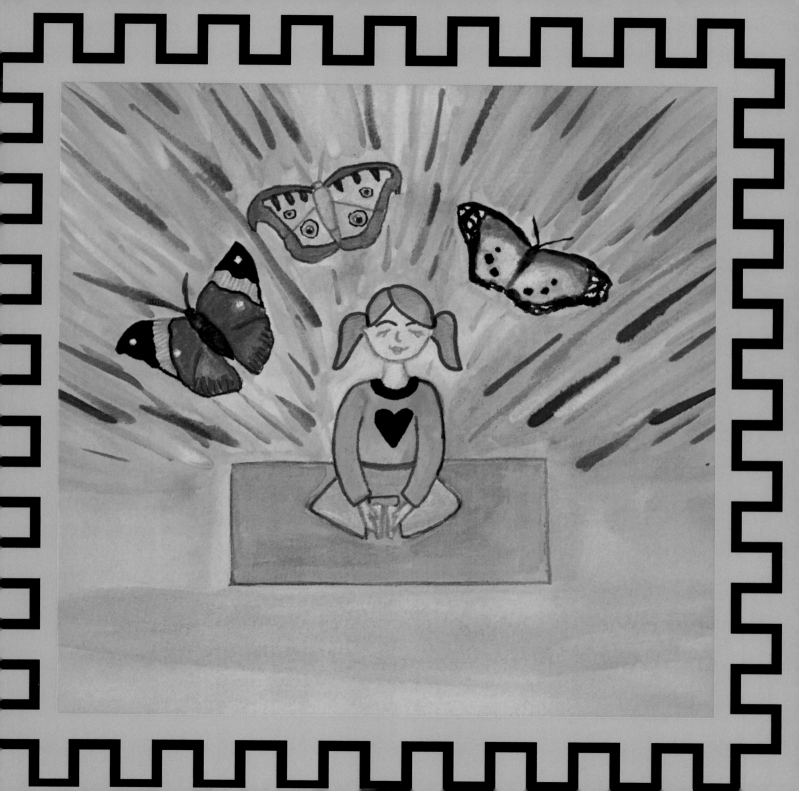

Guided Visualization

As you lay on your mat begin to imagine yourself floating high above the Himalayan Mountains, the highest mountain range in the world. See the tall mountain peaks covered in snow in every direction you look. Bask in the enormity of the mountains. They have been there for millions of years and people who live there depend on them to meet all of their needs. The air is fresh and crisp. The peaks of the mountains are breath-takingly beautiful. Take a moment to breath in the beauty of this mountain range.

Now in your mind drift to the North west corner of India. This is where the Thar Desert is located. What do you imagine the desert would look like? I imagine the whole desert to be sand dunes as far as the eye can see. Breathe in to this image and exhale. Sand dunes are a large part of the desert however, there are also towns where the houses are made of mud with roofs of elephant grass. In the desert people use camels as a mode of transportation. Imagine what it would be like to climb onto the back of a camel. How many humps does your camel have? Envision yourself riding across the Thar Desert on your camel. It is similar to riding a horse but a bit bumpier.

As you ride your camel across the desert, see people in brightly coloured clothing carrying water jugs from a well. They carry the water on their heads back home to use for cooking and cleaning. Feel the heat of the hot desert sun beaming down on your head. It is very hot and dry here. Imagine what you would wear to protect yourself from the heat of the desert. Now as you continue riding on your camel across the desert, imagine a beautiful sunset. As the sun sets behind the enormous sand dunes the air becomes cool. So cool that you would want a sleeping bag to help you stay warm. Envision the sun setting and cooling off the air.

In your mindseye we are now going to visit the city of Agra where one of the 7 New Wonders of the World, the Taj Mahal is located. Take a deep breath in and imagine yourself standing majestically on the banks of River Yamuna, the Taj Mahal symbolizes love and romance. It is an enormous tomb built by the emperor Shah Jahan for his wife who died giving birth to their 14th child. Construction of the tomb began in 1632. He loved his wife so much that he had the Taj Mahal built so his wife could be buried there. Take a moment to envision the Taj Mahal with walls made of white marble, the dome shape of the temples roof, the archway to the entrance. It is truly a wondrous sight. Breath in this image. Even with 20,000 workers it took over 10 years to build. This is one of India's most famous buildings.

It is made of white marble. When it was being built they used more than 1,000 elephants to help transport the materials. Imagine a 1,000 elephants working to carry in the huge slabs of marble too heavy for humans to move. What does the scene look like? Create it in your mind. Breathe in and out and take in all of this truly exquisite building with as many as 28 different varieties of semi-precious and precious stones used to detail the walls and floor. What would it feel like in your body to see such a beautiful building. Breathe in that feeling of awe and amazement.

We are going to travel again to the capital city of India, New Delhi. New Delhi is the largest city in India and the fifth largest city in the world. Imagine what it would be like to be in such a crowded city. There are people and cars everywhere, but that is not all, there are even cows wandering through the traffic. No one seems to mind the cows and do not do anything to stop them from wandering through the traffic of the crowded city. Take a moment to imagine what it would be like to see cows wandering through the traffic. In India many people belong to the Hindu religion and believe that some animals are sacred which is why the cows are free to wander wherever they like.

Imagine what it would be like to wander through the streets of New Delhi see the shops selling shiny tinsel, braids, sequins and turbans. You find a beautiful bracelet in the market. What does it look like. See all of the details of the bracelet, the colour, the texture the shapes, what it is made of. Who will you give it to when you return home? Envision giving it to that person. How does it make you feel to give them a gift? Breathe in that feeling.

Moving in your mind to the southwest of India into the state of Kerala. Things move a lot slower here than in the big city. Most people living here fish or farm. See the fields of rice, tea and spices. India is famous for the spices and tea grown here. There are also many waterways. Imagine you are taking a tour in a covered wooden boat. Most of the people in this area use boats to get around. You may even see a boat full of children on their way to school. Envision what it would be like to ride on a boat to school instead of a bus. Would you dress differently? Would it feel different to travel to school by boat? Breathe in this experience. In Kerala they have good schools. More people can read and write in this part of India that any other region including the big cities. Imagine what it would be like to not know how to read or write. How would that impact your life?

Let go of that image and see the lush green land surrounding you on your wooden boat. There are coconut groves, rice paddies and coconut husks soaking along the edge of the water. Soaking the husks helps to soften them so that they can be made into rope. Imagine yourself weaving the softened coconut husks into a long rope. What would you use the rope for? Breathe in the beauty and tranquility of this area, the slow paced life, the water, the crops.

Now we will travel to northern India and celebrate the festival of Holi. Holi starts on a full moon in the spring. Breathe in the warm spring air and envision the full moon. The celebration begins in the evening with a bonfire. The next morning everyone prepares their coloured powders. Holi is also known as the festival of colour. Imagine piles and piles of coloured powder being sold in the markets and shops. Imagine all of the colours of the rainbow everywhere your look. People throw water and coloured powder at each other, kids squirt coloured water with their water pistols. Getting stained head to toe is all part of the fun. Imagine yourself running through the street throwing water and coloured powder and blasting your friends with coloured water in your water gun. Even the cows get painted with blasts of colour. At noon the silliness ends, people clean up and visit with family, friends and relax.

Feel this sense of joy and silliness run through your entire body and breathe it all in. Then begin to relax again and feel the sense of relaxation run through your entire body. Breathe in and exhale this sense of calm.

Begin to awaken your body. Roll on to your right side using your arm as a pillow. Come to seated criss cross. Hands at centre in prayer position. "Namaste"

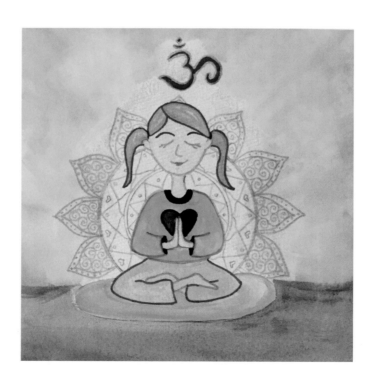

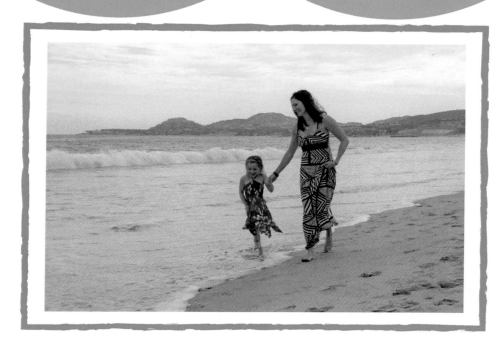

About the Author

Amanda currently lives in Calgary, Alberta with her daughter Ella. They love to go to yoga, travel and go on adventures in the mountains together. Amanda teaches elementary school and has a Masters degree in Education. Her passions are drawing, creating, yoga and reading. She recently started a business called 'Art Mindfulness and Creativity' to help inspire others to find their own creative outlets.

www.artmindfulnessandcreativity.com

27978710R00022